MW00720788

OVER 150 TRULY ASTONISHING BEAUTY TIPS

THIS IS A CARLTON BOOK

Text and design copyright © 2000 Carlton Books Limited
This edition was published by Carlton Books Limited in 2000
20 Mortimer Street, London W1N 7RD

A CIP catalogue for this book is available from the British Library.
ISBN 1 85868 978 3

Printed in Italy

Editorial Manager: Venetia Penfold

Art Director: Penny Stock

Editor: Zia Mattocks

Design: DW Design

Picture Research: Deborah Fioravanti

Production: Garry Lewis

The expression Cosmopolitan is the trademark of The National
Magazine Company Ltd and the Hearst Corporation, registered
in the UK and USA and other principal countries in the world and
is the absolute property of The National Magazine Company
and the Hearst Corporation. The use of this trademark other than
with the express permission of The National Magazine Company
or the Hearst Corporation is strictly prohibited.

Picture Credits The publishers would like to thank the following
sources for their kind permission to reproduce the pictures in this
book: Getty One Stone / Jerome Tisne 13, Andre Perlstein 97;
Sandro Hyams 5, 21, 27, 30, 37, 43, 51, 56 -7, 63, 71, 81,
86, 93, 104; Retna Pictures Ltd 102.

OVER
150
TRULY
ASTONISHING
BEAUTY
TIPS

JAN MASTERS

CARLTON
BOOKS

Original Skin

1

Be skin smart.
STOP trying to categorize your complexion as oily, dry or combination and start treating it as unique and ever-changing. Skin is affected by many factors – it may be drier when you've been flying, more oily in hot weather, or prone to break-out when you're stressed. Assemble a few key products that work for each of your needs and use them *flexibly* – in the same way that you would a capsule wardrobe.

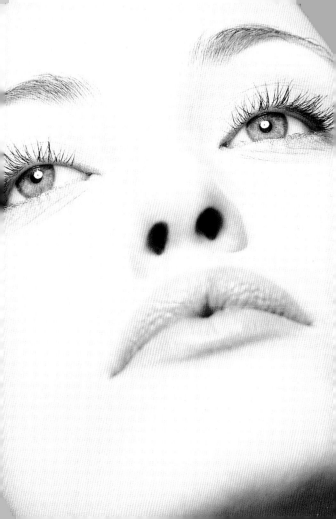

2

New thinking from dermatologists: water-soluble cleansers are the best. The reasons? Water re-hydrates the skin, doesn't drag or pull at it (unlike wiping off cleanser with a tissue) and removes every last smidgen of gunk and grime. Get splashing!

3

Leaning forwards and supporting your face in your hands for a minute or two provides the ideal amount of pressure on **facial skin tissue** to banish puffiness.

It's so tempting, isn't it? That zit is just asking to be zapped. But try to postpone the picking. Unless a spot gives under very gentle pressure, you're simply going to make matters worse. What's more, professional make-up artists insist that an untouched blemish is easier to cover – yup, a comforting thought, models get spots too.

'Scrubbing is for floors,' warns top US dermatologist Patricia Wexler MD. Pass up ultra-scratchy scrubs and scouring pads for daily de-griming and use a good, old-fashioned flannel – it's one of the best skin-loving exfoliators there is. **Note:** buy a white one so that you can throw it in the washing machine whenever you're doing a hot wash.

6

Go easy on the moisturizer: slathering it on all over can be a real skin sin. The should-you-shouldn't-you test: wash your face with a gentle cleanser and then wait **half an hour** to see whether your skin produces enough oil to make it feel comfortable. Target wherever it feels tight.

7

Hold that scalpel.
Research shows that
people who practise
transcendental meditation
have, on average, a 15 per cent
lower level of ageing free-radical
activity. **Ommmmm ...**

**Feast on fresh fruit and vegetables
every day,** and as the juice dribbles
down your chin, remember that
you're stuffing yourself with
vitamins A, C and E – nutritional
superheroes that neutralize nasty
free radicals which, if left
unchecked, zip about zapping
your skin's stroke-me suppleness.

Whoa. Don't use soap or astringent to de-grease oily skin – it simply dries out the top layers, sending a signal to the glands beneath to start pumping out more oil. It may sound crazy, but using an oilier cleanser instead can actually calm greasy skin and stop it going into oil-overdrive.

If you want a **cream** that packs a powerful anti-ageing punch, look for one that contains retinol, a derivative of vitamin A. Gentler than prescription-strength Retin A, it helps skin to recoup some of its bounce-back qualities.

Yes, it is possible to reverse the ageing process! But only if you start using an SPF15 on your face every day. This will give your skin's repair mechanisms a chance to undo some of the sun damage you have inflicted on it previously – the combination of years of everyday sunlight and the odd week of intense cooking on blissed-out beach holidays. If, however, you continue to allow the sun's rays to bombard your skin without protecting it, the cumulative damage will outpace your skin's ability to repair itself. Result? Wrinkles.

Research from the **Volvic Hydration Report** reveals that one in five offices has a humidity level as low as the Sahara, and one in ten is as dry as Death Valley. This is why drinking six to eight glasses of water a day is an essential skin-plumping strategy.

If you get the chance to sit in a **steam room** after an exercise session, grab it. Not only is it fantastic for relaxing your muscles, but it also gives your complexion a hands-free facial, coaxing out toxins, melting away stubborn grime and oil, and revving up the microcirculation.

Way to glow!

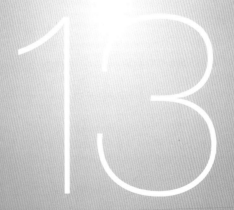

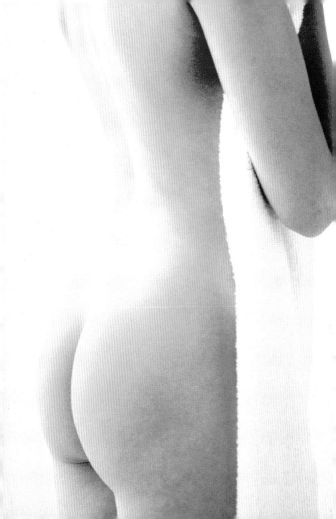

Invest in silk or satin pillowcases. They're more slippery than cotton, so your skin is less likely to be squished into wrinkle-inducing folds.

14 15

Turn your **night-time cleansing** and moisturizing session into a delicious wind-down ritual – massage the back of your neck, scalp and temples; then drench a tissue with a relaxing combination of essential oils and inhale them for a minute or two. We've become so accustomed to a frenetic and frenzied world that we tend to hurry the bedtime routine, but psychologists say that if you focus on personal grooming as precious 'me' time, you'll develop more energy and self-esteem.

Frowning causes furrows, squinting creates crow's feet. A high-tech solution is a Botox injection. This temporarily paralyses the muscles into which it is injected, so no matter how much you screw up your face, the skin over the injection sites stays smooth. The effect lasts for about four months, but because you're not frowning during that time, the skin becomes a little more crease-proof each time you have a treatment.

16

17

You may be able to improve the **water-retentive** qualities of your skin by boosting its production of natural oils called lipids. How? Essential fatty acids (found in Evening Primrose or Starflower oil capsules) are said to promote lipid production, so increase your intake and see what happens.

18

Don't over-apply **eye cream** – it causes puffy eyes in the morning. When you apply cream under the eye, simply dab it along the bone that forms the socket ... and no further. The cream will migrate upwards, providing just enough nourishment to moisturize the skin but not so much as to inflate the problem. Goodbye panda eyes.

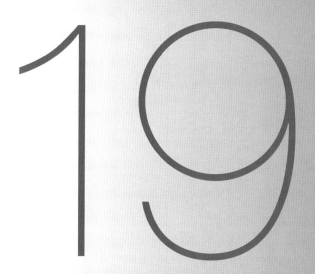

Night-time is the right time to apply treatment creams, according to LA dermatologist Dr Howard Murad. When your head hits the pillow and your mind goes to play on the bouncy castle of dreams, repair mechanisms kick in and cell activity triples. Night creams can boost this process, so don't skimp.

20

There are fewer **sebaceous glands** in your neck than in your face, which is why the skin there can become dry and crepey. To help compensate for this, smooth face products *downwards* and body products *upwards*.

21

Body brushing is the all-over skincare routine that boasts the all-time biggest payoffs. It stimulates the lymphatic system and leaves skin super-soft. Keep the body brush dry and, starting at your feet, work up the body using firm, rhythmic strokes; brush in one direction only and always work towards the heart.

Follow the lead of **top models** shooting on location on far-flung shores (with no beauty counters in sight). Make a body scrub by mixing sea salt with enough

22

olive oil to make it squishy and then adding a squeeze of lemon juice. The salt exfoliates, the oils moisturize, and the lemon juice evens up skin tone and whitens nails. Your skin will feel like a peach that's been dipped in honey.

23

Turn your shower into **DIY hydrotherapy.** Hold the shower head 15 cm (6 in) away from your forehead and mist it lightly. Increase the pressure to massage your neck, back and shoulders, and zigzag a softer spray up and down your legs before directing a harder jet at the soles of your feet. Finish with a cool rinse. Aahhh.

Make-up Shake-up

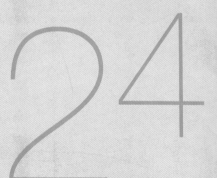

24

The all-time make-up rule from the pros. For maximum impact with a modern twist, play up one feature only – lips or eyes.

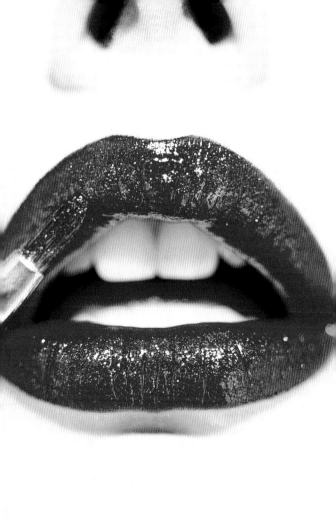

Professionals use **foundation** like concealer, applying it only where it's needed – usually under the eyes, around the nose and on any areas of high colour. When your skin needs all-over assistance, however, dot base onto your nose, chin, forehead and cheeks, and then use *both* hands to smooth the base towards the edges of your face.

A must-learn rule: you cannot, repeat, *cannot* target tiny blips and blemishes by applying concealer directly from a chunky twist-up tube, or from a palette with your fingertip. Use a small brush. Slightly over-apply the concealer and then tap off any excess with your ring finger until you achieve perfect coverage. Now, spot the spot. Bet you can't.

Different shades of concealer do different jobs. You probably already use a lighter shade of concealer than your skin tone for dark areas, such as under-eye shadows, but with puffy areas such as eye bags, the trick is to use a darker concealer (a non-shimmery, liquid bronzer will do) to make them recede. Easy does it though, we're talking teeny-tiny amounts.

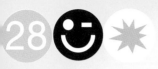

You can take years off your face by concealing the little downward lines at the corner of your mouth. Alternatively, you can just **smile non-stop**.

Take **blusher over the brow bone** as well as the cheeks to give balance to your overall look. Before you brush it on, apply some translucent powder, which will anchor the colour to your skin without any patchiness.

30 When you're looking for the right **shade of bronzer**, go for the colour that you'd turn if you were toasting in Tahiti. For blusher, go for the shade you sport after a hot shower, a winter walk or a steamy session under the duvet.

Position your mirror so that you are facing daylight squarely. If you take the easier-on-the-ego route and apply make-up in a more flattering light, you run the risk of slapping on too much colour and ending up with a scary orange face. For the evening, a mirror surrounded by bulbs, or a vanity mirror with an integral light, is best. A light source that comes from one side only, or above your head, casts shadows that are tricky to work with.

That **very expensive lipstick or mascara** has 'buy me' written all over it. Should you weaken? Studies show that when you go for little-rich-girl purchases, you're making positive statements to yourself:

1 I deserve this expensive item.
2 I will have the means to make myself happier if I have it.
3 I will bring some of the magic associated with this luxury item into my life.

Need any more excuses?
Think not.

Copy the pros. Before applying eye make-up, dust masses of translucent powder under your eyes. When the job is done, simply flick away the powder. All the specks of eye make-up that would have clung to your foundation will be brushed away too.

3334

If you bend your **mascara brush** into a crescent shape (and it will still fit into the tube), it will help you reach the base and tip of every single lash.

If, when you remove the wand from your mascara, it no longer makes a slight slurping sound, it's **time for a new one**.

3536

If you want **wide-awake eyes**, try a trick that top make-up pro Kevyn Aucoin used on Gywneth Paltrow – apply white liquid shadow to the inside corners of the eyes and blend slightly. Who needs sleep?

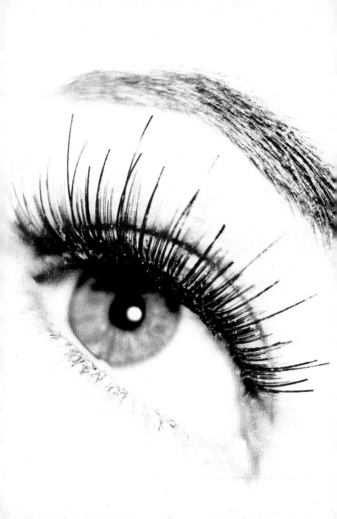

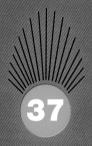

37

Fake lashes are fabulously fun and flirty but they always need to be customized. Trim them to fit the width of your eye, or just use small sections or individual lashes. Make eyes look rounder by adding a few extra lashes to the centre of the lid or 'lift' the eyes by placing lashes on the outer corners. Squeeze a line of glue onto the back of your hand, or a piece of paper, and dip the fake lashes lightly into it to avoid a sticky situation.

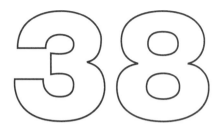

Be an eyeliner know-all ...
For wide-set eyes, place the emphasis
on the inner corners of your eyes.
For close-set eyes, play up the outer
corners and keep the inner corners clear.
For deep-set eyes, lighten the upper lids
with pale shadow and apply liner to the
bottom lash line only.
For small eyes, avoid black liner – try grey,
bronze or chocolate instead. And keep the
line fine – never thick – along lower lashes
only and add upturned tails.

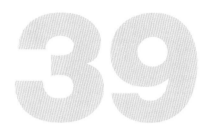

For **eye-smouldering oomph** without having to draw a line at all, dot liquid liner between lashes at the roots.

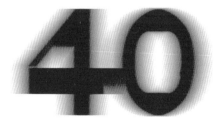

For an instant **lipstick sealant**, prick a vitamin E capsule and slick it over your lip colour.

The shape of your half-used lipstick tells
you whether you're applying it correctly.
If it's ...

Flat, you're applying it too hard to the
lower lip. If you're then pressing your lips
together to transfer colour to the other lip,
the top line will lack crispness.

A sharp slope, you may be holding the
lipstick too vertically. In time it will be at
such a steep angle that it will be hard to
achieve a good outline on the bottom lip.
Turn the lipstick around regularly.

A pyramid, it's a good sign that you're
holding the lipstick at an angle and
applying the colour evenly to both lips.

42

You don't have to give **your complexion** an all-over powder treatment. In fact, for a more modern look, step back and consider which bits you want to matt down – your nose, perhaps – and which bits you want to keep glossy – like the tops of your cheeks, which look more gorgeous with a bit of gleam.

43

Metallics are always hot news, not just for the face but for the body too. But do you go for a gold glimmer or a silver shimmer? The colour code is easy. If you have pale skin (think Nicole Kidman), select silver; if you're more olive-skinned (Salma Hayek), strike gold.

Hair Rehab

Take your lead from the stylists who work backstage at the catwalk shows and break all the rules by concocting styling-product cocktails. What's yours?

• To make wavy hair straight, mix a small dab of conditioner with a larger blob of gel before running it through the hair and blow-drying – the conditioner will stop the gel making your hair crispy, while the gel gets rid of fluffiness.

• To give straight hair a tousled look, mix glossing serum with a squirt of hairspray in the palm of your hand (at close range hairspray turns into liquid). Work it through your hair, scrunching as you go – the spray gives hold, the serum separates.

• To give curly hair more definition, mix gel with serum in equal parts – the extra hold of the gel and the shine from the serum is a real booster for curly hair.

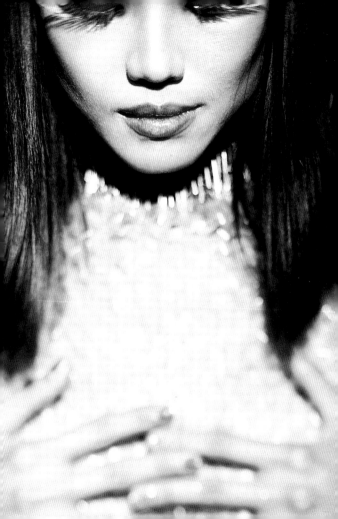

45 Only apply **shampoo** to the scalp – the lather that floods through the length of your hair as you are rinsing is just the right amount to cleanse it perfectly without over-stripping the drier ends. Conversely, apply conditioner to the ends of your hair first, before using what's left on your hands to work through the rest of your hair towards the scalp area. This way you won't over-condition the roots, which tend to need less moisture.

46 Maintain the **muscle** of your styling products by applying it to half-dry rather than sopping wet hair – that way you don't dilute it.

Jumping in the tub before you go out somewhere special? Run the cold water first – it will prevent clouds of steam from wrecking your style.

47

Top TV hairdresser Andrew Collinge shares this quick trick for a too-good-to-be-true shine. Work a small amount of intensive conditioner into towel-dried hair, put on a shower cap to hold in the heat, and let your hair 'sweat' for at least five minutes. The heat will open up the cuticles, allowing the conditioner to penetrate and do its gloss-boosting stuff.

48

Blow-drying only starts to make an impression at 'the conversion point', when hair is turning from damp to dry. Up until that moment you'll be giving yourself arm ache for nothing. Better either to let it reach that stage naturally or rough-dry it with the dryer until it's just damp. And if it becomes too dry while you're still styling, mist it with a water spray.

The average blow-dry fails to look like the pro version because most people get bored and give up before each section is really, *really* dry. 'It's the last minute or two that counts and if hair isn't totally dry, you've wasted all the time you've already spent on it,' warns Nicky Clarke. It's really worth going the extra minute for that **just-stepped-out-of-the-salon finish**. If you do, no one will know you've just stepped out of your bedroom.

If you want to avoid that **'oh-no-I-think-I-hate-it'** feeling as you leave the salon, take a picture (or four) of the style you're after. If you want proof that it's not naff, Sally Hershberger (creator of the famous Meg Ryan cut) confirms that brought-in pics really help. 'A good stylist will be able to say whether the style you love will work on your hair,' says Sally, 'and if not, they'll be able to suggest a viable alternative.'

Do inches matter? Hair that just reaches your bra strap at the back is the sexiest length – according to 43 per cent of men.

Listen to your stylist – they know what your hair type can handle. But if you don't feel fantastically excited about the suggestions on offer, do not be BULLDOZED, be

BRAVE!

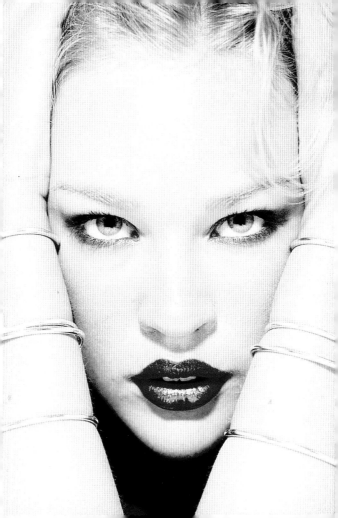

'When you're styling your **hair at home**,  remember to check out the back and sides,' says top stylist Peter Forrester. 'It's all too easy to take ages making sure your reflection in the mirror looks just right and forget everyone else is actually looking at the whole three-dimensional you.' Clue: It's all done with mirrors.

If you think you want to go lighter, hunt out 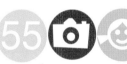 some of those cute pictures of you as a toddler – the chances are that your hair was lighter then and the colourist can copy those tones for the most complexion-flattering colour. It's the shade that nature gave you, so **it's bound to work**.

Crack the colour code ... 56
Rich red tones flatter
pale and creamy ivory skin. Blonde looks
sensational with light golden skin tones.
Dark brown and black enlivens sallow,
yellow-based complexions.

Don't wash your hair 57
just before a re-colour –
not only do roots show up better on
unwashed hair, grubby locks are easier to
handle too. Not *too* grubby, obviously.

Get off your **guilt trip** about spending money on your hair – why are you dithering about paying £80 for highlights when you would probably dish out £200 on a special outfit without blinking? Your hair creates just as much of an impression as clothes – and you'll wear it more – guaranteed.

Want to make a really striking change to your hair without lopping loads off the length? **Ask for a fringe** – it's the instant image-morpher most frequently requested, and great for narrow and long faces too.

Mussed up, playfully unfussy hair is seriously sexy. 'It's sensual because it shows you're fearless enough to appear undone,' says New York's hot hairdresser John Sahag. Heavily textured or razor-cut hair is the easiest to mess with. Simply whack in some wax and use your fingers to coax in that just-rolled-in-the-sack sexiness. Be warned – a brush is a no-no because it will knock out the texture. How easy is that?

With miles of aisles of fancy, schmancy styling products from which to choose, which ones do you take to the check-out? Top stylist **Damien Carney** says, 'Choose one product to help you cope with wet hair and one to give your hair shape and hold when it's dry – that way you'll have something to suit your hair type and style.'

Broken up with your boyfriend? Stop yourself before you go for a drastic cut. Maybe you could go for a blunter, edgier version of what you already have – it may be all you need to feel that bit more pulled together. Or try adding complexion-enhancing highlights or lowlights. Leave the re-style for when you're feeling more upbeat ... or, even better, for when you've found a new lover.

62 63

Do you always come out of the salon feeling your cut is average rather than out of this world? If the answer's yes, find a stylist who will your cut hair when it's dry. **Michael Van Clarke** (Nicky Clarke's brother) is a great exponent of dry-cutting; he feels that it's easier to see (and account for) the individual quirks of your hair when it's dry, especially if it's wavy or coarse-textured – which can look deceptively similar to poker-straight hair when it's wet.

Hair may look dull because it is bored with its long-standing relationship with your shampoo. Research shows that staying loyal to one lather can actually have a detrimental effect on hair, as it becomes immune to the shampoo's benefits. Solve this by varying your hair's routine. It's also worth ditching that favourite works-wonders shampoo a few weeks prior to a big occasion and then switching back to it a few days before.

64

If you want fabulous, **born-again hair** for big occasions, book up appointments with your hairdresser well in advance to avoid disappointment, even if you'll be having your usual style. Make them for at least a week ahead of the event because it's when hair grows that zillionth of an inch after cutting that it looks just right.

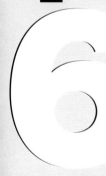

Date Night

Here's a secret tip for **full-on eyeliner** that lasts the distance, from top make-up pro Vincent Longo. 'Stroke on pencil liner first, then apply a little dark eyeshadow as powder liner over the top to help to set it, and then finish with a line of liquid liner,' says Longo. It'll be there until lunch time – tomorrow!

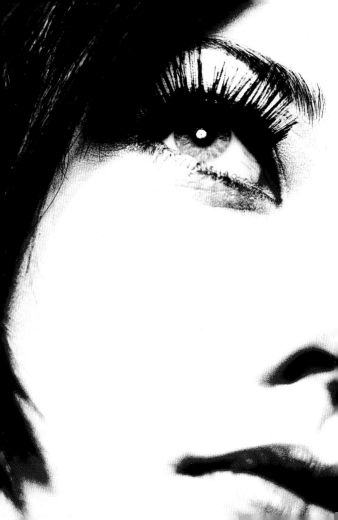

Women **who wear lipstick** kiss more – bare-lipped babes pucker up 20 times a week, while lipstick-lovers smooch a sexy 60 times.

'Red lips are **bold and sexy**, full stop,' says Fiona Fletcher, make-up artist to the likes of Jennifer Aniston. If you're a virgin scarlet starlet, start by using ultra-sheer reds and work your way up to traffic-stopping vermilions. 'But don't make the Cupid's bow too perfect – it can be a touch too Minnie Mouse. Knock the peaks down a bit for a more rounded, luscious result,' advises Fiona.

'Bright lipstick is the make-up equivalent of high heels,' says top make-up artist Daniel Sandler. Use a nude liner first to seal the edges and stop the colour bleeding, and then fill in with **lipstick** using a brush. 'But when it comes to eyeshadow, naked is sexy.' Using a neutral shade looks clean and confident, and it lets the lipstick zing out – emphasis should come from a streak of eyeliner and lashings of mascara.

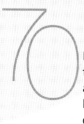

Make your cosmetics work over-time. Add a cream highlighter along the collarbone for a lustrous sheen, extend blusher down the cleavage and then brush shimmer on the rounded tops of the breasts.

For Bambi lashes – there's absolutely no getting away from it – you need to call in support from an eyelash curler. Position curlers at the base of the lashes and squeeze gently for a few seconds before opening and removing. Try to get it right first squeeze, as second attempts often cause strange kinks. Then you need lashings of mascara – but don't wait for each coat to dry, it just causes clumping.

Blend a pale yellowy blusher on top of a pinky shade to soften the edges into a sexy blur. It has the same face-flattering effect on your skin as candlelight.

Celebrity manicurist **Kristi Marie Jones**, whose clients include Jennifer Lopez and Courtney Love, suggests using a metallic varnish as a base coat and topping it with a bright but translucent shade for a nail colour with more sparkle and depth. Her favourite combo? Pinky mauve metallic and see-through scarlet.

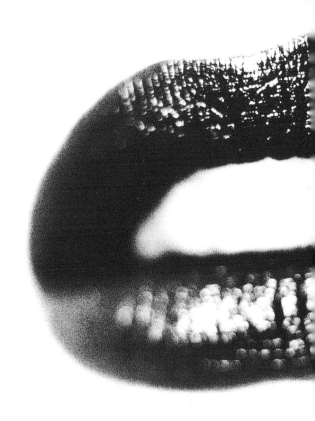

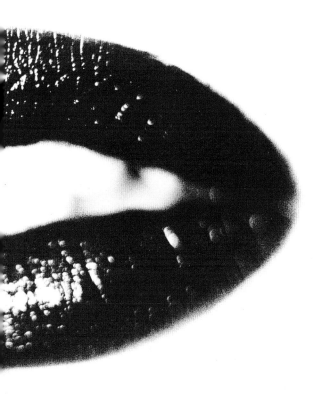

74

For the softest, **most kissable lips**, slough off dry flakes with a flannel while you're taking a hot, steamy shower or bath.

The easiest way to achieve hair with **slept-in sexiness** is to do it for real. The night before your date, work a dab of wax through your hair and add a few plaits, then just ruffle it out in the morning.

75

76

There's nothing sexier than an **all-over tan** and with fake tan you can cover every last inch. Exfoliate, moisturize and then apply fake tan as you would any body lotion. Really rub it in for even coverage but go easy on ankles and knees, which tend to absorb colour faster than other areas. And the best tip of all? Wear very thin plastic disposable gloves when you're applying it. Deeply unsexy, but then again, so are orange hands. When you strip them off, put a tiny amount of self-tan on the back of one hand and rub the backs of both hands together.

Take time out for a **deep and delicious bath** before a hot date. Make-up pro Olivia Chantecaille says, 'I love masses of bubbles and essential oils in the bath. I lie back and convince myself that all my stress is dissolving into the water and disappearing into every last bubble.' Spookily, it works.

'**Clean hair** is sexy hair,' says top hairstylist Sam McKnight. 'Make sure your hair and scalp are freshly washed so that when your boyfriend leans over to kiss your head, he'll be knocked out by the fabulous scent of your hair.' Greasy roots tend to pick up grime quickly, so if you don't have time to wash your hair, use a dry shampoo and mist with fragrance.

According to Joachim Mensing, a psychologist working in the fragrance industry, you should have a **shower or bath** a couple of hours before going out for maximum sex appeal – you'll still feel fresh but your own smell will have started to come through. Only then should you apply fragrance – it will merge with the smell of your own skin, upping its sensuality quotient.

80

Time: 11 pm. Destination: **Far-flung beach**. Departure date: Tomorrow. Problem: Huge pile of suncreams, sandals and sarongs plus five-speed hairdryer all to be crammed into one suitcase. Panic stations. To avoid this scenario, start collecting luxury travel-size pampering treats and free samples well before you plan to jet off. And check with the hotel which items are provided – maybe you won't have to lug that hairdryer after all.

81

As for make-up, think desert island, says make-up artist Barbara Daley. 'A summer holiday is the one time of the year you can count on a healthy glow so it's always best to keep your **make-up simple**.'

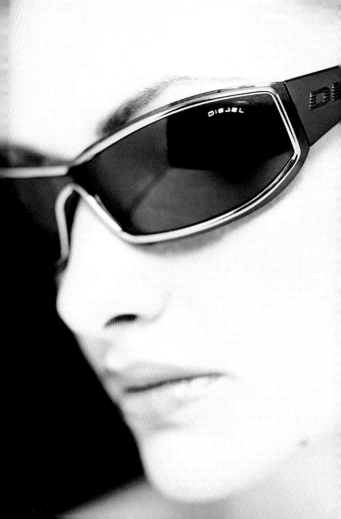

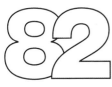

Stow all beauty and medical items in transparent zip-top bags – it cuts down on nerve-fraying rummaging. Pack wash stuff in your hand luggage – if your suitcase goes AWOL, you'll be so glad you did. But don't decant pills into anonymous bottles – you might want to check your recommended dose and customs may want to be able to see that it's a prescription drug.

Banish any bafflement as to the difference between **UVA and UVB** protection now – A is for ageing rays and B is for burning rays. The star rating, usually found on the back of the bottle, identifies UVA, while the SPF, dealing with UVB, is always on the front. It's the SPF number that is the most important to check because it's the burning UVB rays that can cause the most damage to the long-term health of your skin.

84

Understand your **highs and lows**. SPF60s are good for extremely sun-sensitive skin but ultra-high factors don't screen out significantly more rays than traditional high factors such as SPF25. If you want to see the maths, SPF15 screens out about 92 per cent of UVB while SPF30 screens out 96 per cent.

85

When it comes to SPFs, 2 + 2 doesn't equal 4. Using an SPF15 on your face and adding a foundation with an SPF5 doesn't give you a coverage of SPF20, for example. Your **protection level** will only ever be that of the highest factor you are wearing.

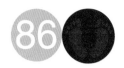

Crash tanning gets you nowhere – quite apart from being dangerous, it's a waste of time. The colour you'll be sporting after two weeks will be much the same as if you had speed-tanned early on. This is because much of the colour of a quickie tan is actually redness as the skin starts to burn (even if you don't feel you're burning). The colour of your tan is genetically programmed – fast or slow, you'll be the same colour in the end.

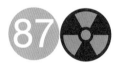

Use fake tan before you fly off on holiday for total confidence at that first hit-the-beach-and-drop-the-towel moment. Self-tan also helps to disguise unattractive cellulite. Big bonus.

According to a study at Harvard University in the US, there is one ingredient in fake tan called **dihydroxyacetone** (DHA) that can protect skin against ageing UVA rays by absorbing them. It's not effective against UVB – the dangerous burning rays – so you'll still need a suncream with a high SPF.

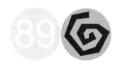

Get the measure of **suncream**. Apply about a teaspoon of suncream to your face – you're spreading it too thin if you use any less than this and that will knock down your SPF15 to about an 8. For your body, you'll need a 200 ml (6.8 fl oz) bottle for each week you're on holiday – at least!

Be a **water babe** with brains and remember that the sun's rays can penetrate fairly deep water, so swimming or splashing about doesn't protect you from the sun – the reverse, in fact. Wet skin burns more quickly than dry skin, so take extra care post-dip. What's more, chlorinated water washes off suncream faster than sea water so, if you're by a pool, always apply waterproof suncream regularly and reapply after towel-drying.

Hand on heart – and on hips – cellulite creams can only help if you're prepared to exercise more, eat sensibly, and drink more water and less alcohol. Then again, a butt-beautifying regime has top-to-toe payoffs. All the above will also give you a come-alive complexion and more stamina.

Amino acids in oily fish stimulate the metabolism and aid the process of lipolysis (breakdown of fats). You can also help reduce fatty deposits with a diet high in complex carbohydrates and low in refined sugars.

Fluid retention makes cellulite look worse. Paradoxically, drinking more water will help – aim for 1–2 litres (1½–3½ pints) a day.

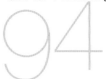

Jonathan Goodair, personal trainer at London's Home House club, suggests this pre-holiday butt-blasting exercise:

1 Lie face down, with your head resting on your hands.
2 Breathe in and slowly lift one leg off the floor, hold for one second, breathe out and lower it.
3 Keep the exercising leg straight with your foot pointed and try to focus on lengthening it (your hips shouldn't lift at any time).
4 Perform 10–20 slow, controlled repetitions per leg. Do this every day during the month before your holiday.

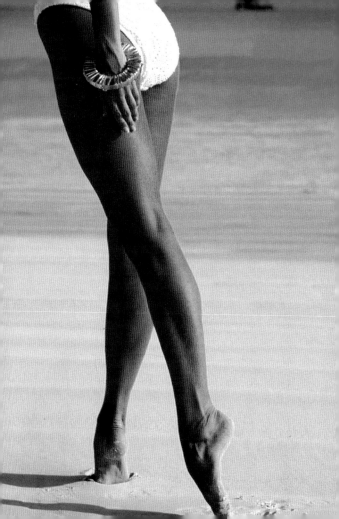

For tousled texture, rub a dab of serum into sea-damp hair – while the salt gives a mermaidy texture, the serum will give gloss and protection.

Brush bronzer onto cheeks but don't forget brows, chin and nose to mimic the places where the sun naturally hits your face. Apply pinky blusher over bronzer for an even more realistic-looking tan – it gives an extra hint of sunny warmth.

Is **sun protection** for your hair really necessary? Absolutely. UV rays break down the hair's protein structure leaving it dull and weak. And colour fades because the hair shaft tends to swell, which allows chemical colour molecules to escape.

98

Summer humidity can make your hair act out of character. Curly or processed hair, which is more porous, absorbs moisture from the air and goes frizzy. Solution? Twist and pin it up to minimize surface area, or use serum which coats the hair, creating a humidity barrier. Straight, fine hair can't absorb the moisture from the air so it lies on the surface and tends to make the hair look lank. A chunky cut with heavy layers on top and shorter ones underneath will support the style – and a blob of volumizing mousse worked through will help.

Incorporating different disciplines into your regular fitness regime – running, weights and yoga, for example – ensures that your body uses a far wider range of muscles than it does if you stick to a constant routine. And when you're on holiday, you should exercise on the sand – it makes you work twice as hard (and exfoliates your feet, too).

According to **Tomas Maier**, who spent ten years designing swimwear for Hermès, you should invest in two swimming costumes – one dark, for the start of your holiday, and a lighter one for when you have a tan.

Dye your eyebrows as well as your hair. Tinted brows that nearly match your hair will really dramatize your eyes – but always ask a pro to do it. Get your lashes dyed too, then you can toss away your mascara with confidence and avoid emerging from the pool looking like something from *The Rocky Horror Picture Show*.

Go on – **treat yourself** to a pre-flight manicure and aromatherapy massage. Ask for a blend of lavender and eucalyptus oil – it can help your immune system deal with bug-laden, recycled cabin air.

What's the most **flattering way to lie** when you're posing for a holiday snapshot by the pool, sipping your Tequila Sunrise? According to Brenda Venus, a stylist for *Playboy*, you should lie on your side, cross one leg over the other and bend your legs slightly inwards towards your body. It makes your hips rise and your waist narrow.

Glam up your suntan lotion. Wende Zomnir, founder of Urban Decay Cosmetics, crushes up shimmery bronze eyeshadow and mixes it into suncream for added shimmer.

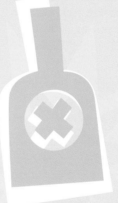

Top hairdresser **Charles Worthington** says that a pre-holiday re-style is better than a post-holiday chop. The reason? You won't be left with any white lines around your hairline where the sun's rays didn't reach. Nicky Clarke agrees that it's best to cut before you run – not only will your holiday image be crisper, your hair will be better able to deal with hot sun and salt water.

105

106

If your skin tends to look shiny shortly after you have applied your foundation, mix a drop or two of toner with a little base in the palm of your hand – it has a noticeable **grease-decreasing effect**.

Run dry of spot-cover? Use the foundation that collects around the neck of the bottle – it will be slightly thicker because the air has got to it, and it will be the perfect match for your skin tone.

107

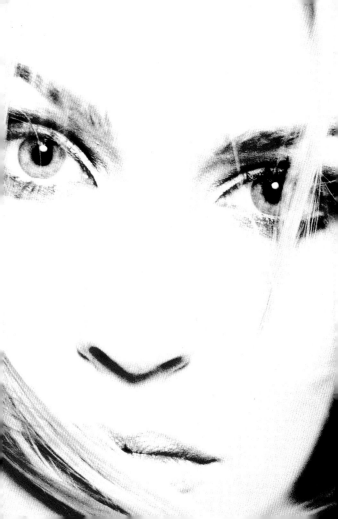

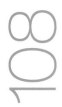

To remove **static from hair**, run a fabric-softening tissue right down the length from the roots to the ends. Alternatively, smooth on a dab of face cream.

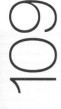

If you're going out in the evening straight from work, there's no need to remove all your make-up and start again. Simply spritz with a water spray and blot with tissue, then use cotton buds to clean up under the eyes. 'But don't add new foundation on top, it tends to cake,' says Ruby Hammer, co-creator of the Ruby & Millie cosmetics range. 'Dot a shimmery bronzer onto the skin instead and blend it in with fingers for a quick-as-a-flash glow.'

If **virgin colour** is peeking through at the roots, but you haven't got three hours to spend flicking through *Hello!* at the salon – hide re-growth with a temporary touch-up. Try coloured brow gel or hair mascara (even ordinary mascara will do).

Been clubbing ... no time to wash your hair the following morning? Charles Worthington reckons that the golden rule is not to brush. Even if your hair isn't greasy, the dirt and smoke that it's picked up will make it look that way if you smooth it down by brushing. Spritz it with a blow-dry spray instead, tip your head upside down and blast with a hair-dryer. For curly hair, mist with detangling spray and finger-style.

112

If you have **dry hair**, swap your cotton pillowcase for satin or silk versions – they don't absorb natural oils.

113

For **uneven lips**, use frosted white eyeshadow and draw a fine line along the area you want to fill out – it catches the light and creates the illusion of a larger outline.

114

If you want to shrink a **seismic smacker**, steer clear of glosses and go for darker lipsticks instead. Alternatively, if you want to use a more neutral or paler colour, use a lipliner *inside* the natural lip line, before filling in your lips and then blending with a matching lipstick.

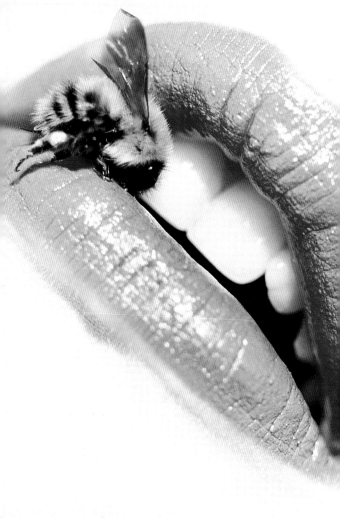

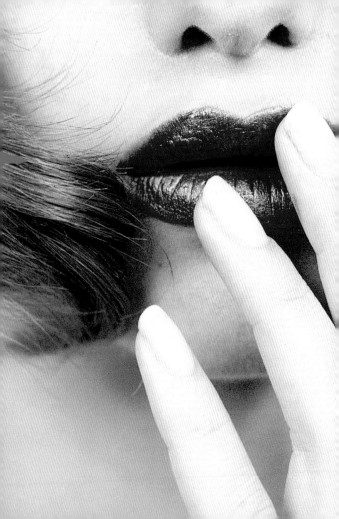

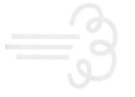

Forget **blowing** on your nails to dry them – dipping them in icy water is much more effective.

116

If your **nails are short**, try a 'squoval' shape – in between an oval and a square. It emphasizes the length but, because you're not filing them down the sides, it makes the nails stronger. Top tip: the abrasive strip on a matchbox will serve an emergency file.

117

Sweet almond oil massaged into nails makes them stronger and more supple, but the key is a little and often – keep one bottle by your bedside and another on your desk at work and use it as an alternative to worry beads.

A mane maintenance trick from **supermodel** Kirsty Hume ... For the ultimate once-a-month conditioning, saturate hair with jojoba oil and leave it for 30 minutes, before washing it out.

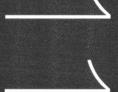

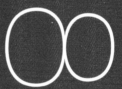

For an instant curl booster, pour boiling water into a bowl and scrunch your hair over the **steam**.

119

When your **curling tongs** are on the blink or your heated rollers are playing it cool, simply scrumple up pieces of aluminium cooking foil into long sausage-shapes, wind sections of hair around them, bend the ends over to secure them and blast with a hairdryer. The foil will heat up, building in body and curl. Now, that's what you call throwaway technology.

Raid the kitchen cupboard. For super-shine, apply a mashed banana, combined with 1 tablespoon of sunflower oil 30 minutes before shampooing. Perk up a flagging perm by rinsing the hair with 1 teaspoon of lime juice in 0.5 litres (1 pint) of cold water before washing (the citric acid ups the bounce factor by contracting the inner cortex of the hair shaft).

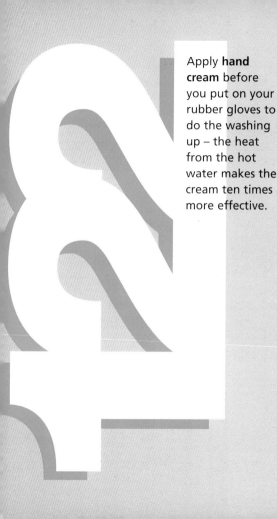

Apply **hand cream** before you put on your rubber gloves to do the washing up – the heat from the hot water makes the cream ten times more effective.

123

Apply a **fresh top coat** of polish to a new manicure every other day – it will look pristine for almost ten days. If you run a little polish along the cut end of the nail, it will seal the colour and prevent chipping as well.

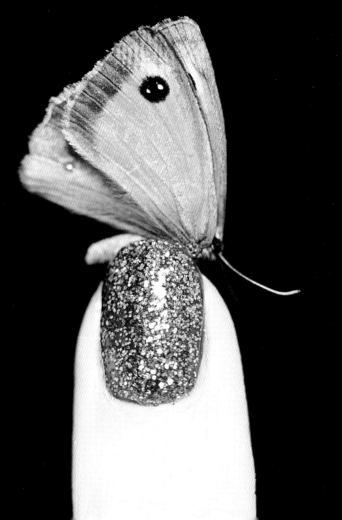

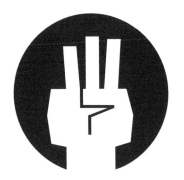

124

Do three things at once – comb on a deep conditioner, spread on a face pack and have a moisturizing soak – a time-saving and performance-enhancing strategy because the steam from the bath helps make the pack penetrate faster.

125

To take the brassy tones out of dyed-blonde hair, top hairdresser Daniel Field suggests smothering your head in **tomato ketchup**. Apply it to dry hair and leave for 30 minutes. Eating chips at the same time is optional. Then rinse and shampoo.

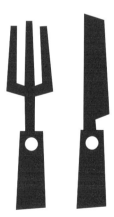

Spa-licious Treats

Heat treatments such as saunas, steam rooms and Jacuzzis are perfect before a massage because they warm up the muscles. The therapist can then work your stress knots with gusto.

127 Take jewellery off before you go into the sauna – it will heat up very quickly and can **burn your skin**.

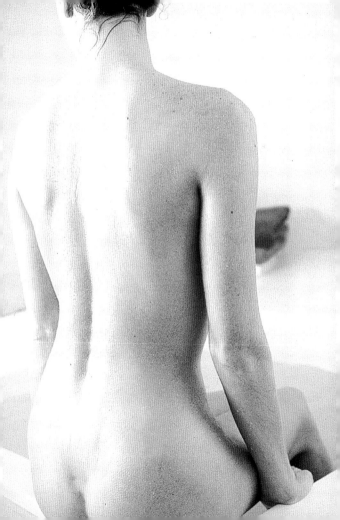

All-over body scrubs are the best bet as your starter treatment. It whisks off dead skin cells and allows any lotions and potions applied during your stay to really sink in and get working.

Raising the **body's temperature** by taking a sauna or sitting in a steam room or Jacuzzi does more than relax you and help the skin eliminate toxins – it has also been found to strengthen the immune system dramatically.

Plan **aromatherapy sessions** as your last treatment of the day. You want the oils to have plenty of time to sink into your skin and perform their magic – if you follow them with swimming or water treatments, all the good work will simply be washed away.

Thalasso-what? Thalassotherapy is a form of water therapy that uses sea water and seaweed extracts in a variety of different treatments to rev up the circulation and detoxify the system. Seaweed- and mud-wraps make you sweat it out, blitz showers are invigorating and underwater massages melt away tension.

Meet your knead. Arm yourself with knowledge about different massages so that you don't find yourself in the position of wanting to be stroked … when you're getting pummelled.

Aromatherapy: Essential oils are blended to suit your individual needs and the therapist works in smooth, soothing strokes. Perfect for de-stressing.

Swedish: Involves long, broad, firm strokes with plenty of kneading and friction. Excellent for knots, aches and pains.

Tui Na: A Chinese massage that's very physical for both you and the therapist (it's almost like one-to-one personal-fitness training). The aim is to release muscular and skeletal tension.

Thai: An ancient therapeutic massage that incorporates yoga-like stretching, gentle rocking and pressure-point work. It can be relaxing or stimulating.

One of the latest ways to **remove hair** permanently is with red and infrared light. How does it work? When the light penetrates the skin, the hair shaft and follicle, which contain more pigment than the surrounding skin, absorb more light. This causes the temperature within the hair follicle to rise, with the result that the hair cell degenerates and dies. Although it is non-invasive, a patch test is always recommended to see how your skin reacts.

Shopping for a facial? Talk to the therapist first and be very clear about the problems you want to blitz. A deep-tissue massage will stimulate the lymphatic system and is good for alleviating puffiness; an aromatherapy facial can help calm sensitive skin; a micro-peeling or exfoliating facial will polish dull, flaky skin; and for anti-ageing, you may want to try a facial that includes the use of electrical micro-currents, which aim to stimulate tissue repair.

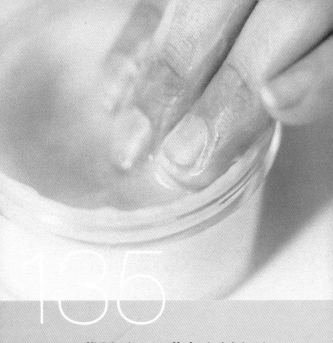

135

It's official. The payoffs for indulging in **beauty treatments** are more than skin deep, according to Horst Rechelbacher, founder of Aveda. Experts now realize that if you consciously cram some extra me-time into your schedule, you start to feel more powerful and in control of your life. So ask for a facial … and hey, make it snappy.

Don't be afraid to speak up at any time if you don't feel comfortable during a treatment, whether you're overheating in a herbal wrap or caught in a cold draught during a massage. Spa treatments are about personal pampering not endurance, but it's amazing how many women who wouldn't hesitate to state their case at work suddenly become tongue-tied when they're wrapped in a towel.

Pre-pay for manicures so fumbling with cash doesn't **smudge your polish**.

Most **spa treatments** require a fair amount of stripping off – although you can usually retain a thong during massages and wear your bikini for water treatments. Tell your therapist what you'd be most comfortable wearing and then try to relax. They're very good at strategically covering you with folded towels at all times. And hey, they have seen it all before!

Scentsory Pleasure

Proof that a **fragrance** can provide a man with a snapshot of your sensuality comes from one of the world's greatest perfumers, Jean-Paul Guerlain. 'When I'm travelling, I don't carry a photo of my girlfriend – I simply spray her scent, and instantly she's right there next to me, proving perfume is more powerful than any picture.'

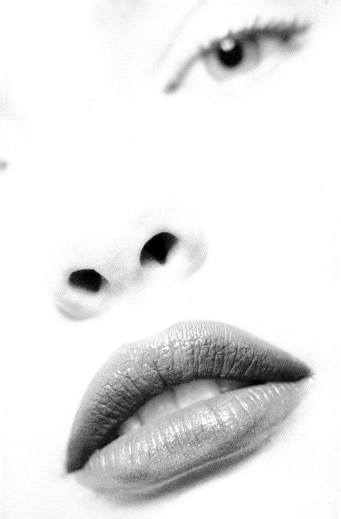

Scent is inextricably linked to memory, so if you're strategic about when your man is first introduced to a new fragrance, he'll forever remember its first-time-out impact. If you lace the early evening anticipation with a new perfume, from that night on, that scent will always conjure up those feelings. For your next trick – use it when you need to twist him around your little finger.

The **science of aromachology** is the blending of aromas to produce specific put-you-on-a-high effects. Want to feel revved up and sexed up? Then make a beeline for jasmine, scientifically proven to stimulate brainwaves. Need to chill-out and relax? Lavender or mint will de-frazzle any stressed-out soul. And just so you don't feel selfish, the effects work on anyone within nuzzling distance, too.

What's the world's favourite passion-provoker? **Vanilla.** 'All around the world it's considered deeply erotic,' says Jean-Paul Guerlain.

143

As your **sense of smell** is directly linked to your memory, one of the easiest ways to make yourself feel at home in a hotel room is to make it smell like home. So if you love to sprinkle essential oils in the bath or spritz the sheets with scent, then do the same in your hotel. That way, when you return each night, you'll instantly provoke that glad-to-be-home feeling.

144

Don't buy a fragrance because you love it on someone else – skin type, diet and the soaps and lotions you use create an individual odour print that influences the way a **perfume develops on your skin**.

145

Keep your **experimentation** down to four scents or less. Test them on your body, placing them as far away from each other as you can to avoid concocting an unidentifiable stew. Make a note of which one is where – it's easy to lose track.

146

Test a fragrance properly by living with it for a day or two – infatuation is world's apart from lasting love.

147

Wearing **scent behind the ears** may be traditional but it's really not the best place for strategic dabbing because secretions from sebaceous glands around your hairline can alter the fragrance's effect. Try other perfume hot spots instead – the front of your ankles, the nape of your neck, the crook of your elbow and – the most powerful pulse point of all – the back of your knees.

148

Lemon and peppermint essences will help you face the day; camomile and lavender will help you wind down in the evening.

149

The most effective scent-carriers are breezes, heat and moisture. So if you spray the hem of a floaty skirt with fragrance on a hot, humid summer's day, your perfume will pack a **powerful punch**.

150

If you can no longer smell your own fragrance when you wear it, it's simply because your nose has got used to it. Don't be tempted to up the dose, because everyone else will be able to smell it quite adequately! Re-educate your nose by switching to the bath products in the same range – the formulation will be different enough to revitalize your **sense of smell**, allowing you to appreciate your fragrance anew.

151 **Deodorants** can clash unattractively with your chosen fragrance – and it's the same story for strong-smelling hairspray. Avoid a struggle for air space by opting for unscented ones.

152 Generally keener than that of men, women's sense of smell is further intensified during **ovulation**. What's more, women produce a scent when they're ovulating that is subliminally attractive to men and even prompts arousal. Maybe you should hold the Chanel No. 5 during those days when nature has you by the nose.